# GREEN SMOOTHIE RECIPES!

## THE WORLD'S MOST DELICIOUS GREEN SMOOTHIE DIET RECIPES

Copyright © 2013 by Ivy Martin
All rights reserved. This book or any portion thereof may not be reproduced or used in any manner whatsoever without the express written permission of the publisher except for the use of brief quotations in a book review.

Printed in the United States of America.
First Printing, 2013

Salem Fox Press
www.SalemFox.com

# TABLE OF CONTENTS

- Introduction ............................................. 2
- Pineapple Passion .................................... 5
- Green Goblin ............................................ 6
- Coconut Crush ......................................... 7
- Tropical Titan .......................................... 8
- Melon Monster ......................................... 9
- Pear Pick-Me-Up ..................................... 10
- Cucumber Craze ...................................... 11
- Broccoli Bash .......................................... 12
- Age Defying Avocado ............................... 13
- Dandelion Detox ..................................... 14
- Bok Choy Blast ........................................ 15
- Watermelon Wonder ............................... 16
- Go Go Goji ............................................... 17
- Cherry Grape Chiller ............................... 18
- Perfectly Pear ......................................... 19
- Luscious Lime Twist ................................ 20
- Awesome Arugula ................................... 21
- Green Pepper Goodness .......................... 22
- Green Giant ............................................ 23

| | |
|---|---|
| Coconut Carrot Craze | 24 |
| Strawberry Banana Bonanza | 25 |
| Papaya Mango Madness | 26 |
| Pomegranate Celery Splash | 27 |
| Rad Raspberry Twist | 28 |
| Raspberry Watermelon Wonder | 29 |
| Awesome Apple Rapini | 30 |
| Beet Green Blast | 31 |
| Fresh Fig & Banana | 32 |
| Watermelon Wake-Up | 33 |
| Banana Berry Blizzard | 34 |
| Broccoli Kiwi Bash | 35 |
| Mango Green Tea Madness | 36 |
| Perky Cucumber Pear | 37 |
| Adventurous Apricot | 38 |
| Savory Strawberry Banana | 39 |
| Kombucha Kraze | 40 |
| Luscious Lychee | 41 |
| Mouthwatering Mango Meal-Replacement | 42 |
| Raisin Rocker | 43 |
| Succulent Swiss Chard | 44 |
| Coconut Melon Mixer | 45 |

| | |
|---|---|
| Bok Choy Bliss | 46 |
| Tropical Coconut Cooler | 47 |
| Exotic Elderberry | 48 |
| Basic Berry | 49 |
| Fabulous Fruit Cocktail | 50 |
| Cucumber Pear Pizazz | 51 |
| Parsley Punch | 52 |
| Dragon Fruit Dash | 53 |
| Green Tea Geisha | 54 |
| Island Ice | 55 |
| Kickin' Kefir | 56 |
| Spirulina Splash | 57 |
| Kiwi-Kale Thirst Quencher | 58 |
| Persimmon Paradise | 59 |
| Caribbean Cucumber | 60 |
| Blueberry Boost | 61 |
| Pommelo Plunge | 62 |
| Awesome Aloe | 63 |
| Strawberry Smash | 64 |
| Mango Melon Machine | 65 |
| Lychee Lagoon | 66 |
| Dragon Fruit Delight | 67 |

| | |
|---|---|
| Watermelon Wango Tango | 68 |
| Parsley Peach Fizz | 69 |
| Lychee Lemonade | 70 |
| Hot Hot Jalapeno | 71 |
| Hello Tangelo | 72 |
| Just Dandy Dandelion | 73 |
| Basil Breeze | 74 |
| Grape-Orange Gala | 75 |
| Nectarine Nirvana | 76 |
| Flaxseed Fusion | 77 |
| Mint Mango Magic | 78 |
| Bok Choy Berry Boost | 79 |
| Spinach Sunset | 80 |
| Date Delight | 81 |
| Ginger Berry Blaster | 82 |
| Banana Boat | 83 |
| Carrot Mango Crush | 84 |
| Strawberry Swirl | 85 |
| Almond Apricot | 86 |
| Rich Rapini | 87 |
| Pina Colada Concoction | 88 |
| Apricot Antioxidant | 89 |

- Black Cherry Sipper ..... 90
- Sweet Citrus Sunrise ..... 91
- Creamy Cucumber Apple ..... 92
- Pretty Pomegranate ..... 93
- Date-Orange Dream ..... 94
- Plum Powerhouse ..... 95
- Apricot Appetite Control ..... 96
- Succulent Strawberry Vanilla Soy ..... 97
- Pommelo Perfection ..... 98
- Slimming Strawberry Guava ..... 99
- Tangy Tangerine Twist ..... 100
- Hydrating Watermelon Workout ..... 101
- Early Morning Elderberry Escarole ..... 102
- Raspberry Rhubarb Remedy ..... 103
- On The Go Orange ..... 104

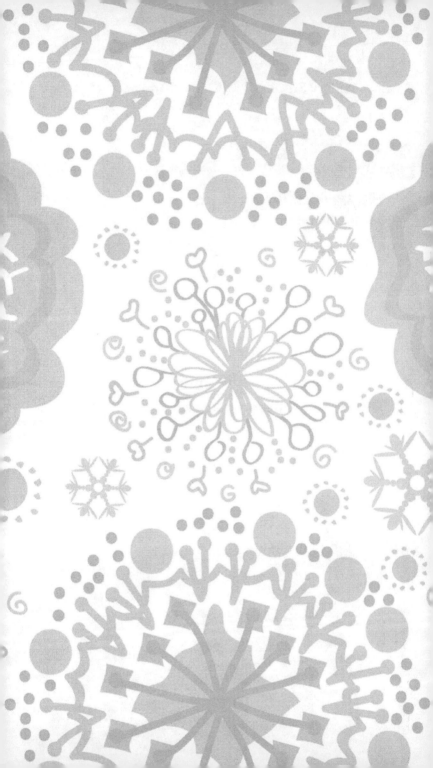

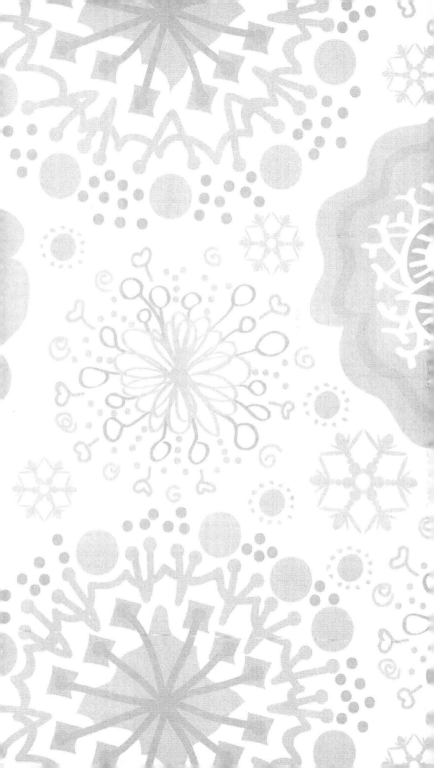

# Introduction

Green smoothies can be powerhouses of nutrition, adding much needed vitamins and minerals to your daily diet. Smoothies contain raw foods, which retain their maximum health benefits. What makes a smoothie "green"? Any numbers of fruits, vegetables, or herbs add the green to each smoothie, including spinach, kale, parsley, chard, green apples, collards, celery, arugula, dandelion and turnip greens to name a few. These are then blended with additional fruits, vegetables, and liquid to achieve a great tasting, healthy smoothie. They are easy to make, and are a great breakfast food or pick me up later in the day. Invest in a travel mug or thermos, and green smoothies make the perfect portable treat.

Green smoothies are full of healthy ingredients, and often contain two or more servings of fruits and vegetables in one serving. They are generally high in fiber, antioxidants, and Vitamins A and C, at the very least. You might be surprised to know that they can also be a good source of protein and iron, depending on which greens you add to your drink. Drinking a green smoothie can help you consume the recommended daily amount of several vitamins and minerals, and are the perfect way to increase your daily intake of vegetables. Many people struggle to consume the daily recommended servings of vegetables, green leafy vegetables in particular. Adding a green smoothie to your daily regimen can make meeting that goal a little bit easier. Added bonus? Kids love them!

If you are looking to lose weight, green smoothies can be your secret weapon. They are low in fat and sugar but high in water and fiber. Green smoothies not only nourish your body, they keep you fuller for longer, and the fiber content

# GREEN SMOOTHIE RECIPES!

helps move waste through your digestive tract. Drinking a smoothie before a meal helps fill you up so that you eat less, without sacrificing nutrition or feeling hungry. The high water content also helps to keep you hydrated. Since green smoothies also contain fruit, their natural sweetness can help curb cravings for sugar and sweets, helping you stick to a healthy eating plan.

Green smoothies can help break caffeine cravings by providing a long lasting energy boost without the crash, anxiety, jitters or nervousness that can accompany caffeine intake. The high nutrition content of smoothies help with mental clarity, and many people report clearer skin and better circulation with regular green smoothie intake. Depending on what health benefit you're looking for, there's a smoothie recipe that's right for you!

Green smoothies are also a great detox food. Free from processed foods, added sugars, dyes, or dairy products, they give your body a break from food that is hard to digest. Removing unhealthy sugars, fats, and simple carbohydrates from your diet can help improve blood sugar levels, reduce inflammation, get rid of headaches, and generally improve your overall wellbeing. A nutritious smoothie can keep a great motivator to help you stick to a weight loss or detox plan because it tastes great and keeps you full.

This cookbook provides all the information you need to embark on your journey to health one green smoothie at a time. While the base of the smoothie is always something green and leafy, the flavor combinations are infinite. Looking for a smoothie to help you lose weight? Increase your intake of fiber? There's a smoothie for you. With additions such as peaches, strawberries, pineapple, blueberries, papaya, and mango just to name a few, it's possible to have a different smoothie every day. By using fruits and vegetables that are in season or that have been flash frozen, it's possible to enjoy budget friendly smoothies

## THE WORLD'S MOST DELICIOUS
## GREEN SMOOTHIE DIET RECIPES

at a fraction of the cost of expensive juice bar smoothies. While ideally consumed immediately, green smoothies can be prepared in advance, and sealed to maintain freshness, making them a great grab and go breakfast. So grab your blender, and get ready to embark on a path to wellness, one green smoothie at a time.

# GREEN SMOOTHIE RECIPES!

## Pineapple Passion

### Ingredients:

3/4 cup green grapes

1 shot wheatgrass juice or 1 packet of wheatgrass powder

1/2 green apple, cored

1/2 cup fresh, cubed pineapple

1 cup ice

### Directions:

Add all ingredients to your blender, cover and blend until smooth. Add filtered water to achieve desired consistency. Refrigerate and serve chilled if desired.

# Green Goblin

### Ingredients:

2 ½ cups fresh baby spinach

1 large handful fresh mint leaves

2 medium pears, cored and cubed

Juice of ½ lime

1 green apple

1 cup ice

### Directions:

Add ingredients to your blender, leaving the greens for last. Blend until creamy. Add filtered water to achieve desired consistency. Enjoy!

**GREEN SMOOTHIE RECIPES!**

# Coconut Crush

### Ingredients:

1 ½ cups fresh baby spinach

¾ cups coconut milk

¼ cup vanilla yogurt

2 medium green apples, cored and cubed

½ cup shaved coconut

1 cup ice

### Directions:

Pour coconut milk, yogurt and shaved coconut into blender. Blend thoroughly. Add green apples, baby spinach and ice, blend again. Add more coconut milk to achieve desired consistency.

THE WORLD'S MOST DELICIOUS
GREEN SMOOTHIE DIET RECIPES

# Tropical Titan

### Ingredients:

3 ½ cups kale

1 cup coconut milk

1 mango, peeled, pitted and cubed

½ cup fresh pineapple, cubed

Juice from ½ lime

1 frozen banana, sliced

1 cup ice

### Directions:

Add ingredients to blender, leaving the kale for last. Blend thoroughly. Add coconut milk to reach desired consistency and enjoy!

**GREEN SMOOTHIE RECIPES!**

# Melon Monster

### Ingredients:

1 cup cantaloupe, cubed

1 cup honeydew melon, cubed

2 cups escarole lettuce

1 cup ice

### Directions:

Add ingredients to your blender, leaving the lettuce for last. Blend thoroughly and add filtered water to achieve the desired consistency.

# Pear Pick-Me-Up

### Ingredients:

2 large pears, peeled, cored and cubed

2 cups fresh baby spinach

1 frozen banana, sliced

½ green apple, peeled, cored and cubed

1 cup ice

### Directions:

Blend all ingredients together, leaving spinach for last. Add filtered water to reach desired consistency. Enjoy!

**GREEN SMOOTHIE RECIPES!**

# Cucumber Craze

### Ingredients:

3 whole cucumbers, peeled and sliced

1 green apple, peeled, cored and cubed

1 cup green grapes

1 cup ice

### Directions:

Add ingredients to blender and blend until creamy. Add filtered water to reach desired consistency and enjoy!

# Broccoli Bash

### Ingredients:

1 large cucumber, peeled and sliced

1 cup fresh broccoli

3 kiwis, peeled and sliced

1 green apple, peeled, cored and cubed

1 cup ice

### Directions:

Chop and steam broccoli until tender. Do not boil or microwave broccoli, or many of the essential nutrients will be lost.

Blend steamed broccoli with other ingredients until smooth. Add filtered water until smoothie reaches desired consistency. Enjoy!

**GREEN SMOOTHIE RECIPES!**

## Age Defying Avocado

### Ingredients:

½ avocado, pitted and skinned

1 cup cubed honeydew melon

1 green apple, peeled, cored and cubed

1 large pear, peeled, cored and cubed

1 cup ice

### Directions:

Blend all ingredients together until smooth. Add filtered water as necessary to reach the desired consistency.

# Dandelion Detox

### Ingredients:

3 cups dandelion greens

2 large pears, peeled, cored and cubed

½ green apple, peeled, cored and cubed

1 frozen banana, sliced

2 kiwis, peeled and sliced

1 cup ice

### Directions:

Add ingredients to blender, leaving dandelion greens until last. Blend until smooth, adding filtered water as necessary to achieve the desired consistency.

**GREEN SMOOTHIE RECIPES!**

# Bok Choy Blast

### Ingredients:

1 ½ cups fresh pineapple, cubed

1 medium head bok choy

1 cup baby spinach

1 large cucumber, peeled and sliced

1 green apple, peeled, cored and cubed

1 cup ice

### Directions:

Place all ingredients in blender, leaving greens for last. Blend until smooth. Add filtered water as needed to reach desired consistency.

# Watermelon Wonder

## Ingredients:

2 cups fresh watermelon, de-seeded and cubed

1 medium bunch fresh parsley (curly or Italian)

1 large peach, cored and cubed

1 green apple, peeled, cored and cubed

½ cup green grapes

Coconut water

## Directions:

Place all ingredients in blender, leaving the parsley for last. Blend until smooth, adding coconut water as needed to reach desired consistency. Enjoy!

# GREEN SMOOTHIE RECIPES!

## Go Go Goji

**Ingredients:**

3 cups fresh baby spinach

½ cup goji berries

2 frozen bananas, sliced

1 green apple, peeled, cored and cubed

Coconut water

**Directions:**

Add ingredients to blender, saving spinach for last. Blend until smooth, adding coconut water until desired consistency is reached.

## Cherry Grape Chiller

### Ingredients:

1 cup pitted cherries (fresh or frozen)

1 cup green grapes

1 cup baby spinach leaves

2 kiwi fruits, peeled and sliced

1 ½ cups ice

### Directions:

Place ingredients in blender, leaving the spinach for last. Blend until smooth. Do not add additional liquid, and enjoy with a spoon!

**GREEN SMOOTHIE RECIPES!**

# Perfectly Pear

### Ingredients:

3 large pears, peeled, cored and cubed

1 large green apple, peeled, cored and cubed

½ cup green grapes

1 cup baby spinach

1 cup ice

### Directions:

Add ingredients to blender, saving spinach for last. Blend until creamy and add water until smoothie reaches the desired consistency.

# Luscious Lime Twist

**Ingredients:**

1 cup kale

2 cups honeydew melon, cubed

1 green apple, peeled, cored and cubed

½ cup green grapes

Juice of 1 lime

1 small handful mint leaves

1 cup ice

Coconut water

**Directions:**

Add ingredients to blender, leaving spinach and mint for last. Blend until smooth, adding coconut water until smoothie reaches the desired consistency.

**GREEN SMOOTHIE RECIPES!**

## Awesome Arugula

### Ingredients:

1 cup arugula greens

1 cup green grapes

2 frozen bananas, sliced

1 cup fresh pineapple, cubed

1 cucumber, peeled and sliced

1 cup ice

### Directions:

Add ingredients to blender, putting in the arugula greens last. Blend until smooth, adding filtered water to reach the desired consistency.

# Green Pepper Goodness

## Ingredients:

2 large green peppers, de-seeded and coarsely chopped

½ cup green grapes

1 large cucumber, peeled and sliced

1 cup fresh pineapple, cubed

1 cup ice

## Directions:

Place ingredients in blender. Blend until smooth, adding filtered water until smoothie reaches the desired consistency. Enjoy!

**GREEN SMOOTHIE RECIPES!**

# Green Giant

### Ingredients:

1 cup baby spinach

1 cup escarole lettuce

1 large cucumber, peeled and sliced

2 green apples, peeled, sliced and cored

1 cup green grapes

2 kiwis, peeled and sliced

1 cup ice

### Directions:

Add ingredients to blender, leaving the leafy greens for last. Blend until smooth, adding filtered water until the desired consistency is reached.

# Coconut Carrot Craze

### Ingredients:

1 cup escarole lettuce

2 large carrots, peeled and coarsely chopped

½ cup unsweetened coconut flakes

1 cup honeydew melon

1 cup ice

Coconut milk

### Directions:

Add ingredients to blender, placing the lettuce in last. Blend until creamy, adding coconut milk until smoothie reaches the desired consistency.

# GREEN SMOOTHIE RECIPES!

## Strawberry Banana Bonanza

### Ingredients:

2 medium heads bok choy

2 frozen bananas, sliced

2 ½ cups fresh strawberries, greens removed

1 red delicious apple, peeled, cored and sliced

1 cup ice

### Directions:

Add ingredients to blender, placing the bok choy in last. Blend until smooth, adding filtered water until smoothie reaches the desired consistency.

# Papaya Mango Madness

Ingredients:

2 cups papaya, peeled, deseeded and chopped

2 mangoes, peeled and deseeded

1 cup pineapple

2 cups baby spinach

1 cup ice

Coconut milk

Directions:

Add ingredients to blender, placing the baby spinach in last. Blend until creamy, adding coconut milk until smoothie reaches the desired consistency.

**GREEN SMOOTHIE RECIPES!**

# Pomegranate Celery Splash

### Ingredients:

2 cups fresh baby spinach

1 cup pomegranate juice

4 large celery stalks, chopped

1 Fuji apple, peeled, cored and sliced

1 cup ice

### Directions:

Add ingredients to blender, placing the spinach in last. Blend until smooth.

**THE WORLD'S MOST DELICIOUS GREEN SMOOTHIE DIET RECIPES**

# Rad Raspberry Twist

### Ingredients:

1 cup pomegranate juice

1 cup fresh baby spinach

1 cup escarole lettuce

2 cups red raspberries

1 cup ice

### Directions:

Add ingredients to blender, placing the lettuce and spinach in last. Blend until smooth.

**GREEN SMOOTHIE RECIPES!**

# Raspberry Watermelon Wonder

### Ingredients:

1 cup raspberries

1 cup fresh watermelon, deseeded and cubed

1 cup escarole lettuce

3 large celery stalks, chopped

1 green apple, peeled, cored and chopped

1 cup ice

### Directions:

Add ingredients to blender, placing the lettuce in last. Blend until creamy, adding filtered water until smoothie is the consistency you want.

## Awesome Apple Rapini

**Ingredients:**

2 cups rapini, chopped

2 green apples, peeled, cored and chopped

1 large frozen banana, sliced

1 cup ice

**Directions:**

Add ingredients to blender, placing the rapini in last. Blend until creamy, adding filtered water until smoothie is the consistency you want.

**GREEN SMOOTHIE RECIPES!**

# Beet Green Blast

### Ingredients:

2 cups beet greens, chopped

1 green apple, peeled, cored and chopped

2 cups green grapes

2 large frozen bananas, sliced

1 cup ice

### Directions:

Add ingredients to blender, saving the beet greens until the end. Blend until smooth, adding filtered water until smoothie is the consistency you want.

## Fresh Fig & Banana

**Ingredients:**

4 large figs

2 large frozen bananas, sliced

2 cups baby spinach

1 cup ice

**Directions:**

Add ingredients to blender, leaving the spinach until the end. Blend until smooth, adding filtered water until smoothie is the consistency you want.

**GREEN SMOOTHIE RECIPES!**

# Watermelon Wake-Up

### Ingredients:

2 cups fresh watermelon, deseeded and chopped

1 cup romaine lettuce

3 stalks celery, copped

1 orange, peeled

1 cup ice

### Directions:

Add ingredients to blender, saving the romaine lettuce until the end. Blend until smooth, adding filtered water until smoothie is the consistency you want.

# Banana Berry Blizzard

### Ingredients:

2 large frozen bananas, sliced

1 cup raspberries

1 cup strawberries

2 cups fresh spinach

1 cup ice

### Directions:

Add ingredients to blender, saving the spinach until the end. Blend until smooth, adding filtered water until smoothie is the consistency you want.

**GREEN SMOOTHIE RECIPES!**

# Broccoli Kiwi Bash

### Ingredients:

1 cup steamed broccoli (can use fresh if you have a high powered blender)

5 kiwi fruits, peeled and chopped

1 green apple, peeled, cored and cubed

½ cup green grapes

1 cup ice

### Directions:

Add ingredients to blender. Blend until smooth, adding filtered water until smoothie is the consistency you want.

## Mango Green Tea Madness

### Ingredients:

1 cup fresh baby spinach

1 cup escarole lettuce

1 ½ cups fresh pineapple, chopped

1 mango, peeled and deseeded

2 large frozen bananas, sliced

Brewed green tea, cooled

### Directions:

Add ingredients to blender, saving the spinach until the end. Blend until smooth, adding brewed green tea until smoothie is the consistency you want.

**GREEN SMOOTHIE RECIPES!**

# Perky Cucumber Pear

## Ingredients:

3 large cucumbers, peeled and sliced

2 medium pears, peeled, cored and cubed

1 green apple, peeled, cored and cubed

1 large handful fresh mint

1 cup ice

## Directions:

Add ingredients to blender. Blend until creamy, adding filtered water until smoothie is the consistency you want.

# Adventurous Apricot

**Ingredients:**

6 apricots, deseeded

1 cup kale

2 pink lady or fuji apples, peeled, cored and cubed

1 large frozen banana, sliced

1 cup ice

**Directions:**

Add ingredients to blender, leaving the kale for last. Blend until smooth, adding filtered water until smoothie is the consistency you want.

**GREEN SMOOTHIE RECIPES!**

## Savory Strawberry Banana

### Ingredients:

1 cup fresh spinach

2 cups fresh strawberries, tops removed

2 stalks celery, chopped

½ cup red raspberries

1 cup ice

### Directions:

Add ingredients to blender, leaving the spinach for last. Blend until smooth, adding filtered water until smoothie is the consistency you want.

# Kombucha Kraze

**Ingredients:**

2 cups romaine lettuce

¼ avocado

2 large frozen bananas, sliced

½ cup green grapes

1 cup ice

Kombucha tea

**Directions:**

Add ingredients to blender, leaving the romaine lettuce for last. Blend until smooth, adding Kombucha tea until smoothie is the consistency you want.

**GREEN SMOOTHIE RECIPES!**

# Luscious Lychee

### Ingredients:

10 lychee fruits, peeled and deseeded

1 cup spinach

1 cup radish greens

1 cup fresh pineapple, cubed

1 cup ice

### Directions:

Add ingredients to blender, leaving the spinach and radish greens for last. Blend until smooth, adding filtered water until smoothie is the consistency you want.

# Mouthwatering Mango Meal-Replacement

Ingredients:

3 cups fresh spinach

2 mangoes, peeled and deseeded

2 large frozen bananas, sliced

½ cup fresh pineapple, cubed

Coconut water

Directions:

Add ingredients to blender, leaving the spinach for last. Blend until creamy, adding coconut water until smoothie reaches desired consistency.

**GREEN SMOOTHIE RECIPES!**

# Raisin Rocker

### Ingredients:

2 cups rapini

½ cup green raisins

1 frozen banana, sliced

1 tablespoon chia seeds

1 cup ice

### Directions:

Add ingredients to blender, leaving the rapini for last. Blend until creamy, adding filtered water until smoothie reaches desired consistency.

## Succulent Swiss Chard

**Ingredients:**

2 cups swiss chard, chopped

2 large frozen bananas, sliced

1 green apple, peeled, cored and cubed

Juice of 1 lime

**Directions:**

Add ingredients to blender, leaving the swiss chard for last. Blend until creamy, adding filtered water until smoothie reaches desired consistency.

**GREEN SMOOTHIE RECIPES!**

# Coconut Melon Mixer

### Ingredients:

2 cups honeydew melon, chopped

1 cup fresh baby spinach

1 cup ice

Coconut water

### Directions:

Add ingredients to blender, leaving the spinach for last. Blend until creamy, adding coconut water until smoothie reaches desired consistency.

**THE WORLD'S MOST DELICIOUS GREEN SMOOTHIE DIET RECIPES**

# Bok Choy Bliss

## Ingredients:

1 cup raspberries

2 large frozen bananas, sliced

1 cup fresh pineapple, chopped

1 cup bok choy

1 cup ice

## Directions:

Add ingredients to blender, leaving the bok choy for last. Blend until creamy, adding filtered water until smoothie reaches desired consistency.

**GREEN SMOOTHIE RECIPES!**

## Tropical Coconut Cooler

### Ingredients:

1 cup fresh pineapple, chopped

½ cup unsweetened coconut flakes

1 large frozen banana, sliced

1 large mango, peeled and deseeded

2 apricots, deseeded

2 cups fresh baby spinach

1 cup ice

### Directions:

Add ingredients to blender, leaving the spinach for last. Blend until creamy, adding filtered water until smoothie reaches desired consistency.

THE WORLD'S MOST DELICIOUS
GREEN SMOOTHIE DIET RECIPES

# Exotic Elderberry

**Ingredients:**

1 cup elderberries

1 cup swiss chard

2 large frozen bananas, sliced

1 cup ice

**Directions:**

Add ingredients to blender, leaving the swiss chard for last. Blend until creamy, adding filtered water until smoothie reaches desired consistency.

**GREEN SMOOTHIE RECIPES!**

## Basic Berry

### Ingredients:

2 cups mixed berries

1 cup fresh baby spinach

1 cup ice

### Directions:

Add ingredients to blender, saving the spinach until the end. Blend until smooth, adding filtered water until smoothie reaches desired consistency.

**THE WORLD'S MOST DELICIOUS GREEN SMOOTHIE DIET RECIPES**

# Fabulous Fruit Cocktail

## Ingredients:

1 cup pears, cored and chopped

1/2 cup cherries, deseeded

1/2 cup peaches, deseeded and chopped

1 cup rapini

1 cup ice

## Directions:

Add ingredients to blender, saving the rapini until the end. Blend until smooth, adding filtered water until smoothie reaches desired consistency.

GREEN SMOOTHIE RECIPES!

# Cucumber Pear Pizazz

## Ingredients:

1 cup pears, cored and cubed

2 large cucumbers, peeled and sliced

4 stalks celery

1 cup turnip greens

1 green apple, peeled, cored and cubed

1 cup ice

## Directions:

Add ingredients to blender, saving the turnip greens until the end. Blend until smooth, adding filtered water until smoothie reaches desired consistency.

# Parsley Punch

**Ingredients:**

1 large handful parsley

1 head escarole lettuce

3 pears, cored and cubed

2 green apples, peeled, cored and cubed

1 cup ice

**Directions:**

Add ingredients to blender, saving the lettuce and parsley until the end. Blend until smooth, adding filtered water until smoothie reaches desired consistency.

**GREEN SMOOTHIE RECIPES!**

# Dragon Fruit Dash

### Ingredients:

2 large dragon fruit

2 large frozen bananas, sliced

1 medium bunch of bok choy

1 cup ice

### Directions:

Add ingredients to blender, saving the bok choy until the end. Blend until smooth, adding filtered water until smoothie reaches desired consistency.

## Green Tea Geisha

**Ingredients:**

2 cups kale

1 pear, cored and cubed

2 cups cubed mango

2 celery stalks

1 cup ice

Brewed green tea, cooled

**Directions:**

Add ingredients to blender, saving the kale until the end. Blend until smooth, adding cooled green tea until smoothie reaches desired consistency.

**GREEN SMOOTHIE RECIPES!**

## Island Ice

### Ingredients:

½ cup unsweetened coconut flakes

2 mangoes, deseeded

Juice of 1 lime

1 cup fresh pineapple, chopped

1 cup kale

1 cup ice

3 tbsp coconut milk

### Directions:

Add ingredients to blender, saving the kale until the end. Blend until creamy. Enjoy!

# Kickin' Kefir

## Ingredients:

½ cup alfalfa sprouts

1 cup plain or vanilla kefir

1 cup baby spinach

Juice of 1 lime

2 cups fresh pineapple, chopped

## Directions:

Add ingredients to blender, saving the spinach and sprouts until the end. Blend until creamy. Enjoy!

**GREEN SMOOTHIE RECIPES!**

## Spirulina Splash

### Ingredients:

1 cup romaine lettuce

2 oranges, peeled and segmented

½ cup strawberries

2 tbsp. Spirulina powder

1 cup plain yogurt

### Directions:

Add ingredients to blender, saving the lettuce until the end. Blend until creamy. Enjoy!

**THE WORLD'S MOST DELICIOUS
GREEN SMOOTHIE DIET RECIPES**

# Kiwi-Kale Thirst Quencher

**Ingredients:**

1 cup kale

5 kiwi fruits, peeled and sliced

1 cup filtered water

1 cup ice

**Directions:**

Add ingredients to blender, saving the kale until the end. Blend until creamy. Enjoy!

**GREEN SMOOTHIE RECIPES!**

# Persimmon Paradise

### Ingredients:

2 fuyu persimmons

2 cups chopped bok choy

2 large frozen bananas, sliced

1 mango, deseeded

1 cup ice

1 cup filtered water

### Directions:

Add ingredients to blender, saving the kale until the end. Blend until creamy. Enjoy!

# Caribbean Cucumber

### Ingredients:

2 large cucumbers, peeled and sliced

1 cup baby spinach

1 cup fresh pineapple, chopped

½ cup unsweetened coconut flakes

1 cup ice

3 tbsp. coconut milk

### Directions:

Add ingredients to blender, leaving the spinach for last. Blend until smooth. Enjoy!

**GREEN SMOOTHIE RECIPES!**

# Blueberry Boost

### Ingredients:

1 cup escarole lettuce

1 cup blueberries

1 cup spinach

2 green apples, peeled, cored and cubed

1 cup ice

1 cup filtered water

### Directions:

Add ingredients to blender, leaving the spinach and escarole lettuce for last. Blend until smooth. Enjoy!

# Pommelo Plunge

Ingredients:

1 pommelo, peeled and segmented

1 cup escarole lettuce

1 cup fresh pineapple, cubed

1 cup ice

1 cup water

Directions:

Add ingredients to blender, leaving the escarole lettuce for last. Blend until smooth. Enjoy!

GREEN SMOOTHIE RECIPES!

## Awesome Aloe

### Ingredients:

1 cup rapini

3 tablespoons fresh aloe vera gel

1 cup green grapes

2 large green apples, peeled, cored and sliced

3 kiwi fruit, peeled and sliced

1 cup ice

### Directions:

Add ingredients to blender, leaving the rapini for last. Blend until smooth, adding filtered water until the smoothie reaches the consistency you like.

# Strawberry Smash

**Ingredients:**

1 cup radish greens

1 cup fresh strawberries

2 celery stalks

2 kiwi fruit, peeled and sliced

1 cup ice

**Directions:**

Add ingredients to blender, leaving the radish greens for last. Blend until smooth, adding filtered water until the smoothie reaches the consistency you like.

**GREEN SMOOTHIE RECIPES!**

## Mango Melon Machine

### Ingredients:

1 cup cantaloupe, cubed

2 large mangoes, peeled and deseeded

½ cup lowfat vanilla or plain yogurt

2 cups romaine lettuce

1 cup ice

### Directions:

Add ingredients to blender, leaving the lettuce for last. Blend until smooth, adding filtered water until the smoothie reaches the consistency you like.

# Lychee Lagoon

Ingredients:

10 lychee fruits

1/2 cup strawberries

1 cup fresh baby spinach

1 cup ice

Coconut water

Directions:

Add ingredients to blender, leaving the spinach for last. Blend until smooth, adding coconut water until the smoothie reaches the consistency you like.

**GREEN SMOOTHIE RECIPES!**

## Dragon Fruit Delight

### Ingredients:

2 dragon fruits

2 large frozen bananas, sliced

1 cup spring mix greens

1 cup green grapes

1 cup ice

### Directions:

Add ingredients to blender, leaving the spring mix greens for last. Blend until smooth, adding filtered water until the smoothie reaches the consistency you like.

THE WORLD'S MOST DELICIOUS GREEN SMOOTHIE DIET RECIPES

# Watermelon Wango Tango

## Ingredients:

1 cup watermelon, cubed and deseeded

1 cup cantaloupe, cubed

1 cup fresh baby spinach

1 cup ice

3 tablespoons coconut milk

## Directions:

Add ingredients to blender, leaving the spinach until last. Blend until creamy.

# GREEN SMOOTHIE RECIPES!

## Parsley Peach Fizz

### Ingredients:

1 handful parsley

1 cup baby spinach

3-4 peaches, deseeded and cubed

½ cup green grapes

Club soda

### Directions:

Add ingredients to blender, leaving the spinach until last. Blend until creamy, adding club soda until desired consistency and fizz is reached.

# Lychee Lemonade

**Ingredients:**

10 lychee fruits

Juice from 2 lemons

1 cup cantaloupe, cubed

1 cup romaine lettuce

1 cup ice

**Directions:**

Add ingredients to blender, leaving the romaine lettuce until last. Blend until creamy, adding filtered water until the mixture has reached the consistency you prefer.

**GREEN SMOOTHIE RECIPES!**

# Hot Hot Jalapeno

**Ingredients:**

1 fresh jalapeno

1 green bell pepper

1 cup escarole lettuce

2 cups honeydew melon

1 cup ice

**Directions:**

Add ingredients to blender. Blend until creamy, adding filtered water until the mixture has reached the consistency you prefer.

# Hello Tangelo

### Ingredients:

Juice from 3 tangelos

1 cup escarole lettuce

1 cup green grapes

2 kiwi fruits, peeled and sliced

1 cup ice

### Directions:

Add ingredients to blender, leaving the escarole lettuce until last. Blend until creamy, adding filtered water until the mixture has reached the consistency you prefer.

**GREEN SMOOTHIE RECIPES!**

# Just Dandy Dandelion

**Ingredients:**

1 cup dandelion greens

1 cup fresh pineapple, cubed

1 green apple, peeled, cored and cubed

Juice of 2 oranges

1 cup ice

**Directions:**

Add ingredients to blender, leaving the dandelion greens until last. Blend until creamy, adding filtered water until the mixture has reached the consistency you prefer.

# Basil Breeze

### Ingredients:

1 cup fresh baby spinach

1 small bunch basil

1 cup watermelon, cubed and deseeded

1 cup honeydew melon, cubed

1 cup ice

### Directions:

Add ingredients to blender, leaving the spinach and basil until last. Blend until creamy, adding filtered water until the mixture has reached the consistency you prefer.

**GREEN SMOOTHIE RECIPES!**

## Grape-Orange Gala

### Ingredients:

1 cup green grapes

1 cup swiss chard

Juice of 1 orange

2 large apples, peeled, cored and cubed

1 cup ice

### Directions:

Add ingredients to blender, leaving the swiss chard until last. Blend until creamy, adding filtered water until the mixture has reached the consistency you prefer.

# Nectarine Nirvana

**Ingredients:**

3 nectarines, deseeded

1 cup baby spinach

1 cup cantaloupe, cubed

1 cup ice

**Directions:**

Add ingredients to blender, leaving the baby spinach until last. Blend until creamy, adding filtered water until the mixture has reached the consistency you prefer.

**GREEN SMOOTHIE RECIPES!**

## Flaxseed Fusion

### Ingredients:

1 cup romaine lettuce

2 tablespoons flaxseed

2 large frozen bananas, sliced

1 cup green grapes

1 green apple, peeled, cored and cubed

### Directions:

Add ingredients to blender, leaving the romaine lettuce until last. Blend until creamy, adding filtered water until the mixture has reached the consistency you prefer.

## Mint Mango Magic

**Ingredients:**

1 small handful mint

2 mangoes, peeled and deseeded

1 cup escarole lettuce

1 cup fresh pineapple, cubed

1 cup ice

Coconut water

**Directions:**

Add ingredients to blender, leaving the romaine lettuce until last. Blend until creamy, adding coconut water until the mixture has reached the consistency you prefer.

**GREEN SMOOTHIE RECIPES!**

## Bok Choy Berry Boost

### Ingredients:

1 ½ cups chopped bok choy

1 cup mixed berries

1 cup fresh pineapple

1 cup ice

### Directions:

Add ingredients to blender, leaving the bok choy until last. Blend until creamy, adding filtered water until the mixture has reached the consistency you prefer.

## Spinach Sunset

**Ingredients:**

2 large green apples, peeled, cored and cubed

3 celery stalks

2 cups green grapes

1 ½ cups fresh baby spinach

**Directions:**

Place all ingredients in blender in the above order. Blend until completely smooth. Add filtered water to adjust the consistency of the smoothie. Enjoy!

**GREEN SMOOTHIE RECIPES!**

## Date Delight

### Ingredients:

¾ cup coconut milk

1 cup halved and pitted dates

1 cup ice

1 cup escarole lettuce

### Directions:

Place all ingredients in blender in the above order. Blend until completely smooth. Add filtered water to adjust the consistency of the smoothie. Enjoy!

# Ginger Berry Blaster

## Ingredients:

1 cup mixed berries

1 knuckle fresh ginger

1 cup ice

2 cups romaine lettuce

## Directions:

Place all ingredients in blender in the above order. Blend until completely smooth. Add filtered water to adjust the consistency of the smoothie. Enjoy!

**GREEN SMOOTHIE RECIPES!**

## Banana Boat

**Ingredients:**

3 large frozen bananas, sliced

1 cup fresh pineapple

1 cup ice

3 tablespoons coconut milk

1 ½ cups kale

**Directions:**

Place all ingredients in blender in the above order. Blend until completely smooth. Add coconut water to adjust the consistency of the smoothie. Enjoy!

## Carrot Mango Crush

**Ingredients:**

3 large carrots

2 mangoes, peeled and deseeded

½ cup pineapple

1 cup ice

2 cups escarole lettuce

**Directions:**

Place all ingredients in blender in the above order. Blend until completely smooth. Add filtered water to adjust the consistency of the smoothie. Enjoy!

## GREEN SMOOTHIE RECIPES!

# Strawberry Swirl

### Ingredients:

1 cup fresh strawberries

½ cup pineapple

1 red delicious apple, peeled, cored and cubed

1 cup ice

1 cup fresh baby spinach

### Directions:

Place all ingredients in blender in the above order. Blend until completely smooth. Add filtered water to adjust the consistency of the smoothie. Enjoy!

# Almond Apricot

## Ingredients:

5 medium apricots, deseeded

1/2 cup almonds

1 tsp. almond extract

1 cup ice

1/2 cup coconut milk

1 cup romaine lettuce

## Directions:

Place all ingredients in blender in the above order. Blend until creamy. Enjoy!

**GREEN SMOOTHIE RECIPES!**

# Rich Rapini

### Ingredients:

1 avocado, deseeded and scooped

1 cup fresh pineapple

1 cup ice

1 ½ cups rapini

### Directions:

Place all ingredients in blender in the above order. Blend until completely smooth. Add filtered water to adjust the consistency of the smoothie. Enjoy!

THE WORLD'S MOST DELICIOUS
GREEN SMOOTHIE DIET RECIPES

# Pina Colada Concoction

### Ingredients:

1 cup fresh pineapple, cubed

½ cup unsweetened coconut flakes

½ tsp. coconut extract

1 cup ice

½ cup coconut milk

1 cup escarole lettuce

### Directions:

Place all ingredients in blender in the above order. Blend until completely smooth. Add coconut water to adjust the consistency of the smoothie. Enjoy!

**GREEN SMOOTHIE RECIPES!**

# Apricot Antioxidant

### Ingredients:

3 apricots, deseeded

½ cup pomegranate juice

1 large apple, peeled, cored and cubed

1 cup ice

1 cup radish greens

### Directions:

Place all ingredients in blender in the above order. Blend until completely smooth. Add filtered water to adjust the consistency of the smoothie. Enjoy!

# Black Cherry Sipper

### Ingredients:

1 cup black cherries, pitted

½ cup strawberries

1 cup ice

2 cups dandelion greens

### Directions:

Place all ingredients in blender in the above order. Blend until completely smooth. Add filtered water to adjust the consistency of the smoothie. Enjoy!

GREEN SMOOTHIE RECIPES!

## Sweet Citrus Sunrise

**Ingredients:**

Juice of 1/2 lemon

2 oranges, peeled and segmented

1/2 cup grapefruit juice

1 cup pineapple

2 cups rapini

1 cup ice

**Directions:**

Place all ingredients in blender in the above order. Blend until completely smooth.

# Creamy Cucumber Apple

### Ingredients:

2 large cucumbers, peeled and sliced

2 large apples, peeled, cored and cubed

½ cup green grapes

1 cup ice

1 cup romaine lettuce

### Directions:

Place all ingredients in blender in the above order. Blend until completely smooth. Add filtered water to adjust the consistency of the smoothie. Enjoy!

GREEN SMOOTHIE RECIPES!

# Pretty Pomegranate

### Ingredients:

1 cup pineapple, cubed

1 cup pomegranate juice

1 cup ice

2 cups baby spinach

### Directions:

Place all ingredients in blender in the above order. Blend until creamy.

# Date-Orange Dream

Ingredients:

3 dates, pitted

2 oranges, peeled and segmented

½ cup coconut milk

1 cup ice

2 cups escarole lettuce

Directions:

Place all ingredients in blender in the above order. Blend until completely smooth. Add coconut water to adjust the consistency of the smoothie. Enjoy!

**GREEN SMOOTHIE RECIPES!**

## Plum Powerhouse

### Ingredients:

4 plums, pitted

1 cup pineapple

1 cup ice

1 1/2 cups radish greens

### Directions:

Place all ingredients in blender in the above order. Blend until completely smooth. Add filtered water to adjust the consistency of the smoothie. Enjoy!

## Apricot Appetite Control

**Ingredients:**

5 apricots, pitted

2 apples, cored and cubed

½ cup fresh pineapple

½ cup green grapes

1 cup ice

1 cup romaine lettuce

**Directions:**

Place all ingredients in blender in the above order. Blend until completely smooth. Add filtered water to adjust the consistency of the smoothie. Enjoy!

**GREEN SMOOTHIE RECIPES!**

# Succulent Strawberry Vanilla Soy

## Ingredients:

½ cup fresh strawberries

½ cup vanilla soymilk

1 apple, peeled, cored and cubed

2 large frozen bananas, sliced

1 cup fresh baby spinach

## Directions:

Place all ingredients in blender in the above order. Blend until completely smooth. Enjoy!

## Pommelo Perfection

**Ingredients:**

1 pommelo, peeled and segmented

Juice of ½ grapefruit

1 cup pineapple

1 cup fresh mandarin orange slices

½ cup coconut milk

1 cup rapini

**Directions:**

Place all ingredients in blender in the above order. Blend until completely smooth. Enjoy!

**GREEN SMOOTHIE RECIPES!**

## Slimming Strawberry Guava

### Ingredients:

2 guava fruits

½ cup strawberries

½ cup pineapple

1 cup ice

1 cup dandelion greens

### Directions:

Place all ingredients in blender in the above order. Blend until completely smooth. Add filtered water to adjust the consistency of the smoothie. Enjoy!

THE WORLD'S MOST DELICIOUS
GREEN SMOOTHIE DIET RECIPES

# Tangy Tangerine Twist

**Ingredients:**

3 tangerines, peeled and segmented

½ cup pineapple

1 cup ice

2 cups rapini

**Directions:**

Place all ingredients in blender in the above order. Blend until completely smooth. Add coconut water to adjust the consistency of the smoothie. Enjoy!

**GREEN SMOOTHIE RECIPES!**

# Hydrating Watermelon Workout

### Ingredients:

1 cup watermelon

½ cup strawberries

2 celery stalks

1 cup ice

1 ½ cups fresh baby spinach

### Directions:

Place all ingredients in blender in the above order. Blend until completely smooth. Add filtered water to adjust the consistency of the smoothie. Enjoy!

# Early Morning Elderberry Escarole

Ingredients:

1 cup elderberries

½ cup pineapple

1 large frozen banana, sliced

1 cup ice

2 cups escarole lettuce

Directions:

Place all ingredients in blender in the above order. Blend until completely smooth. Add filtered water to adjust the consistency of the smoothie. Enjoy!

**GREEN SMOOTHIE RECIPES!**

# Raspberry Rhubarb Remedy

### Ingredients:

½ cup raspberries

½ cup chopped rhubarb

1 large apple, peeled, cored and cubed

1 cup ice

1 cup baby spinach

### Directions:

Place all ingredients in blender in the above order. Blend until completely smooth. Add filtered water to adjust the consistency of the smoothie. Enjoy!

# On The Go Orange

### Ingredients:

2 large navel oranges, peeled and segmented

1 large frozen banana, sliced

2 kiwi fruits, peeled and sliced

1 green apple, peeled, cored and cubed

1 cup ice

2 cups romaine lettuce

### Directions:

Place all ingredients in blender in the above order. Blend until completely smooth. Add filtered water to adjust the consistency of the smoothie. Enjoy!

# GREEN SMOOTHIE RECIPES!

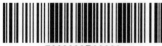

Made in the USA
San Bernardino, CA
20 December 2013